Zing Living
the 4 pillars of health

health & yoga lifestyle with
Young Living essential oils

by Heather Kamala
Wong-Xoquic

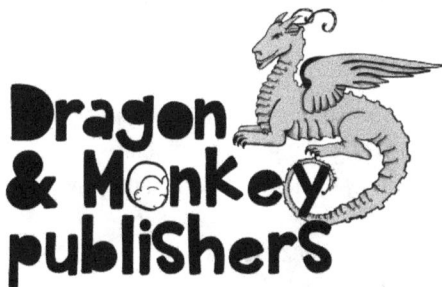

**Dragon
& Monkey
publishers**

San Francisco, California

Published and distributed in the United States of America by Dragon & Monkey Publishers.
Cover design and illustrations: Heather Kamala Wong-Xoquic

Use of images and information about Young Living Essential Oils from www.YoungLiving.com and books by Gary Young. We are distributors of Young Living essential oils and products, member number 2391868.
Young Living membership and products may be purchased at: www.myYL.com/KiDoKids.
All other information, videos and KiDo Kids Yoga or Zing Living products may be purchased at: www.myZingLiving.com or www.KiDoKidsYoga.com.

This is a work of nonfiction. The author of this book does not offer medical advice. The statements in this book have not been evaluated by the U.S. Food and Drug Administration. The product endorsed in this book are not intended to diagnose, treat, cure, or prevent any disease.

Names: Wong-Xoquic, Heather Kamala, author.
Title: Zing Living, the 4 pillars of health,
    health & yoga lifestyle with Young Living essential oils
Softcover ISBN: 978-0-578-41788-2
1st edition, January 2019
Printed in the United States of America

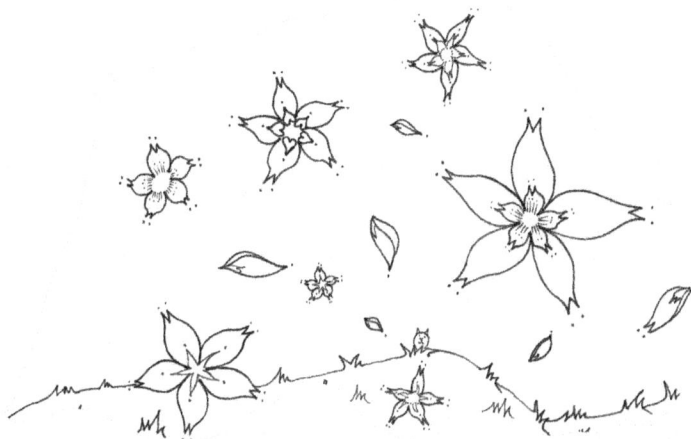

This book is dedicated to
my gorgeous, Mayan husband, Felipe Xoquic,
my compassionate, clever sons, Yaco and Tai,
my master yogi brother, Duncan Wong,
my resourceful, creative parents,
Carol Ma and Victor Wong,
& Gary and Mary Young,
who transformed my
paradigm of health
and wellness.
You all have
made the
difference
in my life,
between
mediocrity
and
greatness.

Table of Contents

Follow us

This Zing Living book is designed to get you started moving towards your best health and wealth. Use the journal pages (throughout the book) and notes (at end of book) for goals, inspirations and ideas that come up while reading and re-reading this book.

Follow the Zing Living lifestyle of health and yoga with Young Living essential oils, purchase your starter kit of oils on our website then subscribe to our YouTube video channel for your new yoga practice, health tips, how to use essential oils in your everyday life to support all body systems and much more. We offer online and live workshops and trainings throughout the year, stay close. www.myZingLiving.com and www.KiDoKidsYoga.com Follow us @myZingLiving @KiDoKidsYoga

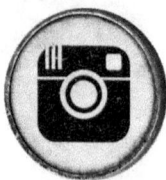

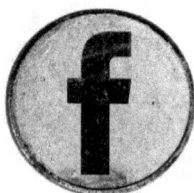

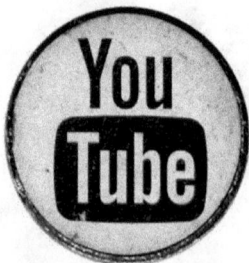

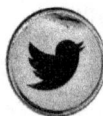

Journaling for Health

We all know that how we feel and how we look are a direct result of what we consume, now let's add to that roster how we act, think and live.

On a Scale of 1 to 10, how do you rate your health? Circle one:

1 2 3 4 5 6 7 8 9 10

Write about your health here.

Rate your health again every 6 months and compare.

Introduction

Welcome to your future, starting right now.
In all of your divine self, you have been guided to this book, this moment. Zing Living is spiraling up from a need for deeper connections to health and nature, to the healing qualities of yoga and the powerhouse support of Young Living essential oils. If you are ready to take action in your life, to uplift your level of health and wealth, then let Zing Living be your guiding force.
Join the Movement! We have lots of products, classes and guidance to get you on your path to health and wealth success. The truth: when you succeed, the whole world becomes a better place. Let's do this!

In this book, I'm going to walk you through how to create the life you most desire. This is what has worked for me, over time, with consistency, kindness, patience and integrity. Creation of your dream life is closer than you think. What does the life of your dreams look like? Is it ultimate health including a rockin' yoga practice no matter your age? Is it building wealth for yourself and others to bring goodness and compassion into the world? Is it bringing yourself to your peak of health? Whatever it be, let this book guide you step-by-step towards your goals. As in life, there are no guarantees, but here, we are going to begin the positive practice of service towards ourselves and others.

'Self Love First' means, we are *not only* fully responsible for our own well being, but when we look into the mirror, there is a profound love of what we see (the whole package). I have learned from my teachers that we are not the ego, we hold the space where greatness can happen. My dearest desire is that this book will inspire you to find the self of your dreams and run with it for the good of the whole, continually taking actions throughout your life in an ongoing spiral upward.

In my KiDo Kids Yoga trainings, I say, "We Lead by Example", meaning we study in depth that which we want to teach. On the certificates we honor our KiDo Kids Yoga graduates with, we quote my brother, Duncan, saying, "Show up. Keep showing up. Find a teacher who inspires you. Drink deeply from that well.

> Would you believe that
> all the worldly glory begins
> with turning the focus inward
> to Loving Yourself Deeply?

I'm going to cover the four pillars that can blast your world wide open, wake you up, and inspire movement:

- Health
- Young Living Essential Oils
- Yoga
- Action

Each of these individually can have profound, life changing effects on you and your communities, and all four together are ridiculously powerful.

Some examples of these four pillars:

• Mind health, as in letting go of the weight of the past and moving forward with lightness and velocity

• Body health, as in creating new habits of healthy eating, drinking and thinking

• A daily yoga practice, incorporating breath, movement and stillness

• Essential oils support from the first and best in the world: Young Living

• Action towards growth, and daily habits of positive movement forward

How fierce are you with your word? In keeping your word. As in, "a warrior of following through with what you have promised, no matter how small or large".

It turns out that a powerful life is cultivated through keeping promises to ourselves and others. It's never too late to implement the changes to transform your habits and lifestyle. This book is your key to that transformation. One baby step at a time towards health and wealth. Consistent actions (no matter how boring) towards your goals over time are the key to creating the life of your dreams.

INTEGRITY = PERSONAL POWER

Journaling for Personal Power

Before we dig into this little book, write about your own level of personal power here, and how you feel currently. As they say in Landmark Education, "there is nothing wrong and there's work to be done."

About the Author

Heather Kamala here, Mama Cat of the KiDo Kids Yoga world, Young Living essential oiler, lover of ink to paper, teacher, dancer, yogi, clown, and designer.
My first successful business, KiDo Kids Yoga preschool, started when my younger son was very little in 1999. Master of Magic by gazing into their eyes with Love and Compassion, I have enchanted generations of preschoolers through to kindergarten including my own two sweet boys. When my husband joined the team, he brought a whole village of influence from his Mayan culture and love of music. We homeschooled our first son and entrusted our second son to our lovely local Waldorf/Steiner school. The Waldorf community fit right into our love of nature, natural life and the cycles of the year we were so familiar with. I love bringing the Old Timey ways into modern life through art, philosophy and my kid's stories.   Our preschool and kid's yoga program are highly influenced by the Waldorf/Steiner philosophies.

I was raised in a family of artists, actors and musicians going back four generations in San Francisco, Chinatown. Rich imagery of China and India created a backdrop of Confucianism, Taoism, the Buddha and Lord Shiva. Yoga and Indian culture were common threads with my Chinese aunties who traveled frequently to India in the 60's and 70's. This greatly influenced my decision to attend yoga classes in the 80's when Swami

Satchidananda was still in his body and Hip Hop blended with Middle Eastern sound was raging in the city. The colors and textures of costume throughout cultures inspired me to become a pattern maker, designer of clothing and accessories, always with historical context.

My father, Victor Wong, raised my brothers and I with total creative freedom. Puppetry, sewing dolls, making toys and always: drawing. He was an excellent stage actor before he became one of the first Asian-American screen actors to break through to Hollywood and the world.

On the flip side, my Lovely English-American mother raised us with 100% natural goodness, which I absorbed totally. From a lineage of carpenters, business owners and upstanding citizens of Washington State, I learned baking, cooking, sewing, gardening and the love of the Great Mother Goddess. Whole foods, supplements, incense and essential oils were common place in our Northern California, pioneer home. The delicious smells and healthful goodness led the way to my future love of Young Living essential oils. When I learned that the founder of Young Living, Gary Young, was a steward of the land and a wonderful gentleman farmer like my great grandfather, I fell in love with Young Living all the more.

Never stopping my love of growth, I continually pursued the healing path of mind, body and spirit. I started my preschool in 1999 and by 2006, I created the global sensation: KiDo Kids Yoga. Now flourishing with families and teachers in America, Europe and Asia. I developed KiDo Kids Yoga as the kid's division of my brother, Duncan Wong's adult system: Yogic Arts and the Yoga Love Warriors (famous for its seven warrior poses). Duncan is known throughout the world as a Master of Movement and Grace with Martial Arts and Ashtanga Yoga.

My third business, Zing Living, is the culmination of all the personal growth, health work and the decades of yoga combined with Young Living. Trust me when I say, integrity is the foundation of my life. I have enjoyed every step of the way with creating Zing Living as a beautiful marriage between health, yoga, essential oils and action.

Being an entrepreneur has been an amazing challenge. I love it and business is growing and flowing, but before all of the success, I had many years of struggle. Years to learn the magical process of how to create something from nothing.
The family mantra is my guiding force in yoga and in business: "Just show up". Just show up on the mat, meaning to develop your personal practice of yoga. Just show up in life, meaning to consistently speak your power and follow through with integrity.

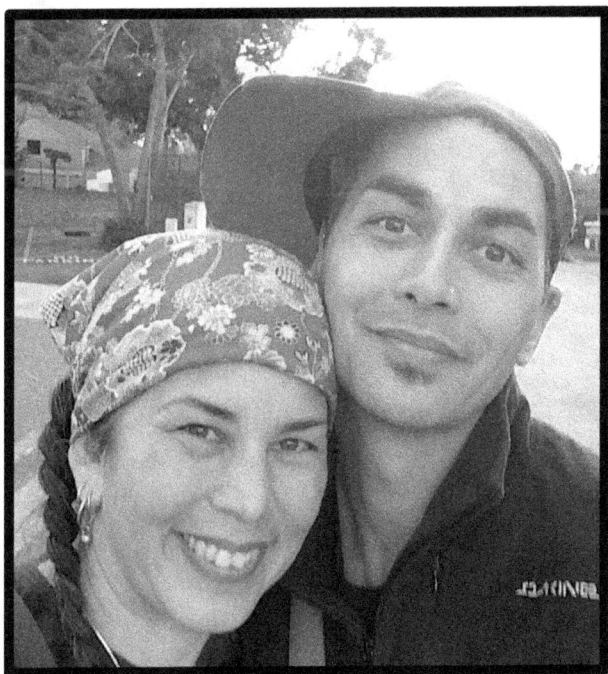
Heather and her brother, Duncan.

HEALTH

Eat, Drink and Live Well

This is the space I choose to create...try it on.
I eat a plant based, whole food diet in a positive life filled with plenty of Young Living essential oils so I can 'oil up' all day long. My electro-magnetic frequency is so high that health radiates from me. I keep hydrated with delicious, pure water and many choices of Vitality™ essential oils. I pray over my meals in private and public. I infuse my drinks with positive vibrations that will expand into the Universe. Can I have that which I desire? Can I take care of my sweet self first? Yes, for the good of the whole!
This is my life and yours if you choose.

One day of what I do and how I think

Morning...
with a drink of water when I wake.

Movement, deep breathing and remembering the dreams that Spirit placed before me as I woke, like bread crumbs to the prize.

Deeply I breath in, slowly I exhale with control as I wake into this gorgeous realm. The place we choose to be, our lives. Breakfast can wait. I'll wait to break that fast, with some stretching to wake up the facia. Some Asana, Pranayama and being present to how my body feels this day. Am I stiff, am I listening to my body and its needs?

Before I get to work, whatever that be today, I'll drink my green or protein smoothie first, then power on as my grandparents did, with integrity and passion.

Is that boring? In my world, that is the peak of cool, the cutting edge of humanity, the highest point we can attain. Why? Because our personal power is sexy and there is no shortcut to building those layers of trust and goodness. I trust myself with myself, my community trusts me with my word. My word is my power. Utmost health begins with the level of integrity that I uphold. There is no guilt or second guessing, I choose every moment to do the right thing, to live well.
Let me explain. As we grow into adulthood, we have the possibility to making powerful decisions as adults. I say this because we all live in different ages throughout our days and weeks. Sometimes, we stand tall to our true age and other times we regress to being teens or toddlers. Ask yourself in a moment of anger or frustration, "How old am I being?" We can choose in every moment to be true to our word and live our full age*.

*from the teachings of the Wisdom Course with Landmark Education™.

When we do, time after time, building the habit of integrity in every corner of our lives as if our lives mattered, that every decision we make matters, our power grows. How can a pebble dropped into the water not ripple?
Can you see that you are the pebble?

We walk with pride and compassion in our Life.
Our cup overflows, we become generous as we achieve abundance in all ways.

Mixed with our yoga life, whole, delicious food, clean water, and health supporting YL essential oils, we become super heroes of possibility.

Afternoon...
Around lunch time, I will eat my veggies and choice of protein. Delicious black beans with cilantro and salsa with two drops of Lime Vitality™ essential oil on organic corn tortillas, so delicious! Or lots of veggies in a salad with garlic hummus, the best! Or a warm lentil soup with scoops of avocado, one drop of Rosemary Vitality™ essential oil and fresh einkorn biscuits, wow! A plant based diet can become a habit. Culturally, across the world, meat and dairy have been comfort foods. Can we ween ourselves from eating animals and their milk? This

is easier when the weather is warm. Would that be the greatest contribution to a global unity and earth saver? Absolutely. We need only take one step, then the other, each time progressing as in a walking meditation.
Think habit as possibility.
Perhaps it is possible to return to a time before animals were farmed. As we are all one, no one species is above another.

Snacktime...
I will pause before a snack to take a quick walk in the afternoon or dance with some pumping tunes or engage my shoulder power for some hand stands. I want my heart to feel loved and taken care of too! Pump it up, heart.
Air is an elemental force, breathe in the goodness, flood the body with oxygen. I keep diffusers with essential oils wafting through the house, reminding me to breathe deeply. Every room can have a different smell depending upon the needs of the moment. The essential oils support the health of all the systems of the body and smell delicious while lifting my spirit.
Drinking water is an excellent way to not only hydrate, but with a few drops of selected Vitality™ essential oils (such as Lemon, Peppermint or Grapefruit) we can enrich the cells, boost the immune system and raise our frequency.

Evening...
Dinner with friends and family? Or dinner alone? Cheers to our good fortune of being full and empty, of being with or without, of non-judgment and self love.

Our lives can be all that we choose. Let us start with Health: strength of mind, power of body and spiritual compassion. From the first cup of water in the morning and the deep breath bridging the connection of dream time to waking reality all the way to the end of our sweet dinner, blessings abound.

As we steer ourselves along the road of life, plucking and digging for that which we crave, I say, wake up, arise greatest self, because we have choices.

I suggest these 10 best practices
for a light giving healthful life...
Cheers to this Ecstatic Life!

My 10 best practices:
- Drink water & Young Living essential oils (Vitality™)
- Practice deep breathing anytime (for longevity)
- Less sugar and wheat intake (find alternatives)
- Eat abundant organic greens and vegetables
- Stretch throughout the day (asana as a lifestyle)
- Complain less (practice gratitude and self love)
- Walk & ride a bicycle more than driving (if possible)
- Laugh long & often (make an effort, be light, let go)
- Forgive others and let go of rage (sweep it away)
- Create a vision board (make lists, keep in action)

Journaling for Health

Write about one of your typical days.
What are *your* best practices?

YOGA

We all have super human powers at our disposal called Yoga! The power to harness the breath and oxygenate the body, the power to change our musculature through consistent, daily movement, the power of the internal clock, the power to tame the mind through quiet stillness and limitless other possibilites.

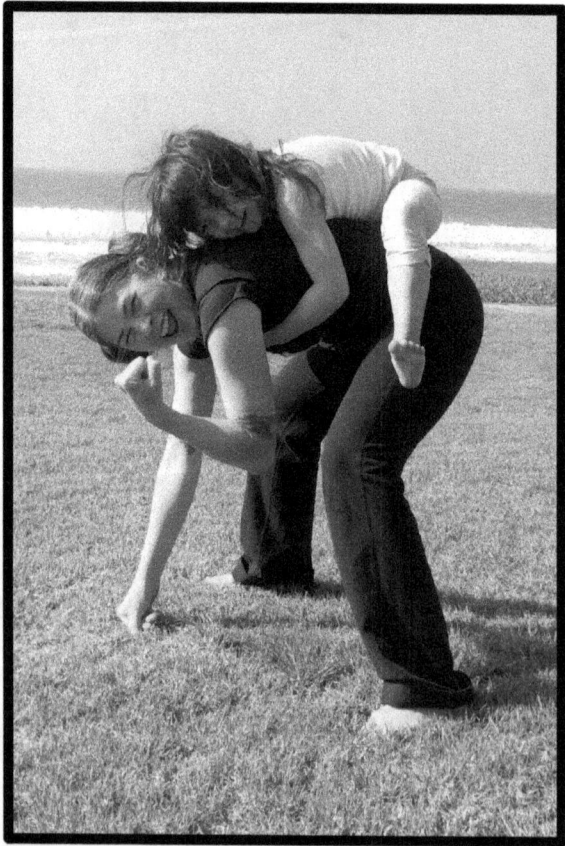

What is Yoga?

To me, it's a natural lifestyle lived close to the earth, close to that which is real. As in the realness of our animal nature. It is a lifetime of study outlined in eight simple branches which guide us to a balanced life. Well known as an exercise program, yoga is actually an ancient way of living from India which has survived throughout the ages and has gained great popularity on every continent as it has passed through each generation. The magical, enlightening quality life takes on when practicing yoga consistently and with pure intentions, has kept it alive for thousands of years.

One of my first yoga teachers, Sri Swami Satchidananda, said that yoga is the science of the mind. The ancient Sage Patanjali, who is the first known scholar to have outlined the meaning of yoga, wrote in his Yoga Sutras circa 5000 BCE:
"yoga is the quieting or stilling of the mind in its changing states".
Here, in the language of yoga, the ancient Indian language called Sanskrit, are the actual words from Patanjali: yogaś citta-vṛtti-nirodhaḥ
योग: चित्त-वृत्ति निरोध–Yoga Sutras 1.2
(yoh-gahs chit-ah ver-rit-tee-hee nuh-roh-dah-ha)
Patanjali's use of the words, "citta vrtti" have been interpreted as the mind chattering without ceasing. Yoga is the quieting of the mind in its changing states or fluctuations. The fluctuations of the mind like waves on a

lake: through yoga we can take control of the constant chattering of the mind and bring peace to our lives. We can watch our monkey mind as a friend from outside, with compassion, but disconnected, detached. How do we bring peace to our minds and lives? Through what Patanjali has outlined in the eight branches or limbs of yoga as the daily lifestyle of:

1) Yamas and 2) Niyamas, how we think and act, how we treat ourselves and others, 3) the movements called Asana or yoga poses, which is key to not only strengthen, but lengthen the muscles and calm the mind, 4) the deep breathing and breath work called Pranayama, which enriches our very cells with an abundance of oxygen, 5) the spaciousness of Pratyahara which brings our practice internally, 6) the extreme focus of Dharana which helps us manifest our dream lives, 7) the deep meditation of Dhyana which cleans our space like a broom sweeping back and forth, and 8) the blissful possibility of Samadhi, that perfect space of mind and body we live towards.

Usually a yoga student begins with Asanas (the physical yoga postures) and Pranayama (breath control) or Dhyana (meditation). As we build our Personal Practice, we may choose to become conscious of how we are living into the other branches, of how free and light we are becoming. Traditionally, yoga, as in martial arts, was taught in a one to one capacity, passing knowledge from teacher to student, from Master to Seeker. Today's yoga dynamic is mostly in a group capacity, trainings and knowledge are even passed down virtually on the internet.

In developing your path of yoga, first recognize the goodness already filling your life. Ponder the lessons already learned from your first teachers: parents, family and friends. Note the areas in your life where yoga already lives. All cultures have beautiful, healthy traditions which make for a society led by conscious human beings. It is our choice of how to live into the expectations of our individual cultures. I always give great reverence to the lineages of yoga teachers from India and beyond. In fact, I was raised by them.

astanga 8 fold path
interpreted for children by Heather Kamala

1	**Yamas**	good living goals
	Ahimsa	be kind, don't hurt others
	Satya	be honest and truthful
	Asteya	boundaries, yours and theirs
	Brahmacharya	self control
	Aparigraha	be generous, not greedy
2	**Niyamas**	myself in the world
	Saucha	keep clean
	Santosha	be peaceful
	Tapas	try hard - have discipline
	Svadyaya	look inside - good habits
	Ishvara Pranidhana	love nature
3	**Asana**	stretch in the pose
4	**Pranayama**	use good breathing
5	**Pratyahara**	control yourself - focus
6	**Dharana**	concentrate in the zone
7	**Dhyana**	be still and quiet
8	**Samadhi**	see your light in nature

The Sanskrit language has reached into our culture with words like: Mantra, Guru and Prana.
The Yoga Sutras are so clearly delineated as to remove the obstacles we find along our paths.

One of my favorite authors, Napoleon Hill, who was a deep philosopher and quite possibly a yogi with the power of the mind, in his last work written in 1938 (Outwitting the Devil), wrote of the virtues of staying on track with positive living and not drifting into a state of 'hypnotic rhythm', like that of a dormant mind or a person without focus.
I say: Awake and Move...You! Let us stay aware and awake in this beautiful life through our practices of health and self love.

My Personal Practice

When I wake up in the morning, I say good morning to the lemon tree, to the lime tree and the sky outside my window. Yes, it sounds corny, but I was raised loving all things equally, and yes, I do believe in fairies.
Before getting out of bed, I say hello to the Spirits who live on my altar, my ancestors and family.
Using the power of the word, I declare out loud,
"I love my life." I started this tradition when, at a low point in my life, a teacher taught me to recite the phrase, "I love my life" upon waking. Even though I didn't feel it at first, miraculously, over time, as I repeated it day after day, I began to feel more empowered and appreciative of my life. It didn't take long to really catch a fire and come true.
The Asana, or stretch, begins right there in bed to wake up the nervous system: forward bends and crunches, back bend over the edge of the bed, then up we go.
Call me wacky, but I don't drink coffee. I wake up with a glass of water that has one drop of Peppermint Vitality™ essential oil that I keep next to my bed, so that no matter how busy life can be, I always drink my water.
After washing up and applying my Melrose essential oil or Tea Tree oil to feet and any skin in need, I practice facial exercises looking in the mirror. Mirror work is a big part of Self Love. I look right at that lady in the bathroom mirror and I love her, all of her. Don't be shy, every day you have the opportunity to love yourself and to greet yourself with a smile in the mirror.

We are not the body or the ego.
We hold the SPACE where it all happens.
We hold the possibility of greatness.

Still in the bathroom, I work out my facial muscles and give my skin some love by rubbing a few drops of Frankincense essential oil to smooth the skin and support my vision. Now here comes the fun part. Pranayama or Breath Control, which is the fourth branch of yoga, and key to building heat that expels toxins and wakes us up. For a double duty pick me up, I use one drop of Peppermint oil on my palm and then I rub both palms together in a clockwise direction (as the Earth moves) three times (thrice round the mountain, as the saying goes) and I make an affirmation. It's a lovely prayer for what I am and what I can be. Yes, I'm pragmatic, but I'm also down with the Spirit. Making a tent over my nose to breathe deeply and evenly, I'm always cautious not to get the oil in or near my eyes or other sensitive skin areas (one drop of Young Living Peppermint essential oil is equal to over 20 teabags). I just breath in and out. Inhaling and exhaling, I count to five slowly on the inhale and again I slowly count to five on the exhale.

Note: in the case that an essential oil causes a burning sensation on the skin or in eyes, never use water, instead rub organic coconut oil or another vegetable carrier oil around the eyes or skin area to calm the sensation.

Next, to juice up and oxygenate, I love my Kapalabhati, or Skull Shining Breath, in which I force the exhale quickly and repeatedly as if blowing my nose on a handkerchief or tissue. Only out of my nose, with mouth closed. According to tradition, it is always best to learn in person from a teacher when possible. As an alternative, you can learn simple Pranayama breath work through our yoga video series on our KiDo Kids Yoga YouTube channel. There we show the complimentary and grounding techniques called "bandha", (pronounced bon-dah) meaning holding or locking a contracted muscle. These are the ancient practices that have been passed down throughout millenia.

Now fully juiced up and ready for my day in just a quick 15-20 minutes, I do my best to make time for another 15 minutes of my Asana practice.
The Asana is the third branch of yoga according to the Yoga Sutras of Patanjali. I have my favorite yoga mat that my brother gave me and there I sit in the morning, with stillness and movement and breath. I listen to my body, sitting with the breath, then to a squat and eventually standing, building heat. I have studied Yogic Arts™ since 2005 and before that Integral Yoga Hatha with Swami Satchidananda's teachers starting in 1987.

practice yoga daily or weekly over a lifetime

I always say, "Any yoga is good yoga". This means even practicing for a few minutes or with children is good for the body, mind and spirit.

Yogic Arts is a lovely form of yoga, created by my brother, Duncan Wong, that focuses on cross core, prana-bandha, wave motion and alignment. Yogic Arts can be practiced with high energy or super mellow.

> **"You need more practice."**
> **~Sung Jin Suh, Master, Kuk Sool Won**

My free flowing yoga practice continues all day long. To honor the circus yogi* in me, I may practice my handstands against a wall or furniture and of course on the mat, balancing. To keep my wrists healthy and support strength, I rub on Copaiba essential oil. To calm any pain, I use Cool Azul® pain relief cream. I love that all the ingredients are from plants. Super old school recipes. Most days I start with sitting poses, then practice my Sun Salutation, that in Yogic Arts we call Warrior Salutation, because we use 7 warrior poses. I end with some core floor work and chanting.

*yogi as in a practitioner of yoga

I've learned that yoga doesn't happen only during a one hour class once or twice a week at the local studio or gym, but all day long, every day. "How often do I practice yoga?" 24/7 is the correct answer. Even while doing my daily chores at home, I will literally hold and stop to get that extra long stretch. Picking up a toy from the floor, ah yes, stretch the back or take a nice standing split. I make sure to do both sides. Squatting down to get something under the sink, ah yes, hold the pipes while you brace your feet for a deep spinal stretch. The list goes on and on.

Patanjali outlined what IS yoga in the Yoga Sutras. My understanding of the Yoga Sutras: the kindness that we show ourselves, our families, and our communities IS yoga. The positive actions we take ARE yoga and the food we choose to consume IS part of yoga.

Journal for Yoga

Look at all of the places in your life where you already see you are living any of the eight branches of yoga. Write about them here.

Imagine your rich yoga life in 5 or 10 years.

Your Personal Practice

If you are new to yoga, I recommend you start your personal practice of yoga in small increments. Always listen to your body. Never do movement that could harm you. Think of your practice as a solid part of your daily life, it should fit your lifestyle. Believe you can practice yoga, no matter your age. Remember, yoga is not just the physical postures and the breath, but the lifestyle of kindness and reflection. Find instructional yoga videos on our KiDo Kids Yoga YouTube channel.

For many years, I thought that because I was over 40, I had reached a limit to the type of yoga that I could practice. I really believed that, until I was encouraged by a teacher to persevere. She pointed out to me how close I was to achieving a hand stand and how great my practice had become since I began adult Asana training in 1987. Armed with the inspiration, I committed myself to mastering the inversions and the arm balances of a Circus Performer, even though I had pain in one wrist. Over time, honoring the pain and giving it space while rubbing it with essential oils and creams daily, as well as taking my supplements such as Agilese™ (with turmeric, frankincense, black pepper, black spruce and more), the strength grew and the pain dissolved. I actually forgot about it. I'm happy to say that at age 50 I attained my first real sense of balance upside down.

Meditation Practices

Find a quiet space where you can be alone, not moving or driving.
Breathe deeply and when you are ready, close your eyes.
Imagine a broom sweeping your concerns away. Every time a thought arises, just sweep it away. Swish to the right, swish to the left, sweep, sweep.
Practice this for just a few moments or for many minutes, as you feel comfortable and inspired to do so. This is a powerful practice for clearing the mind, the first step towards organization.

How often should you clear your mind and when?
- Build a practice of sitting and sweeping the mind everyday for as long as you feel comfortable to do so. Even if your quiet, alone space is in the bathroom, take it without judgement.
- Sweep the mind every time you feel stuck, frustrated, or confused, simply find your quiet space and sweep the thoughts away.
- Breathe deeply while you sweep and eventually open your eyes to see the world fresh again.
- When you go on a walk, sweep the mind as you take each step.
- Practice every night before going to sleep, while lying in your bed.
- Search for creative ways to incorporate the practice of clearing your mind.

Stillness

Stillness as patience, as quiet, as reflection.
Sit in quiet contemplation of nature, the mind will slowly
match the body's stillness. Reflect on nature, on being...

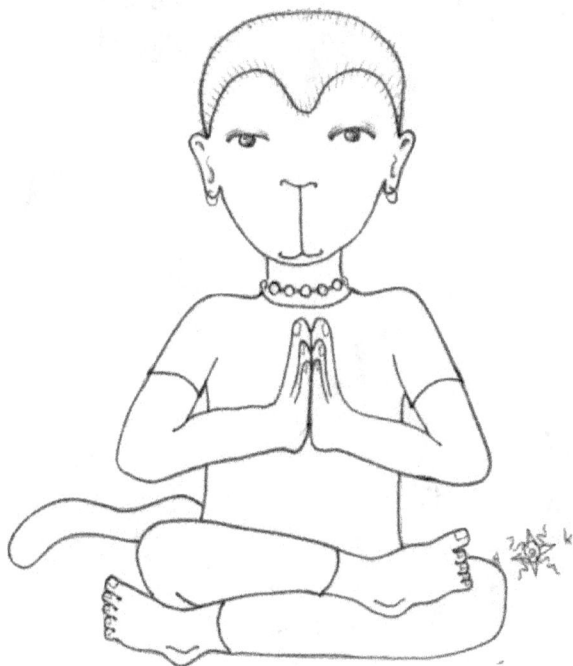

Being in nature helps your Practice. Slowing down to
watch the leaves move in the wind, imagine the tree full
of sweet sap, happy in its being. Following a bird on its
path across the sky, imagine it is content in its flight
going from here to there taking care of its family before
the sun sets.

Bandha Life - Take Your Core Back

Returning to the Sanskrit word: Bandha meaning lock, as in contracting a muscle and holding it in position. When we engage our core (abdominal) muscles, we are engaging our Uddiyana Bandha (oo-dee-ah-nah bondah). Uddiyana in Sanskrit means upward lifting or upward flying. The keyword is Upward with the connection to movement.

I imagine my life constantly gaining momentum in the direction of my dreams, flying ever higher.
I know what your thinking, who wouldn't want that kind of life, but how do we get there?
In Ashtanga (osh-tonga) yoga, when we do our physical practice called Asanas (ah-sah-nahs), as well as our breathing exercises called Pranayama (prah-nah-ya-ma), we hold our Uddiyana Bandha to build heat in the body. Try it, engage your core muscles, shoulders back, chin up! Do this often.
The posture we hold speaks volumes about how we feel. Smile, knowing you have a choice: walk, run or fly.

Now get your essential oils out and breathe in deeply.

Essential oils to support emotional health:
During the 2016 International Grand Convention in Salt Lake City, Utah, Gary Young, the founder of Young Living, spoke about the uses of his essential oil blends to support emotions. To uplift ourselves, physically and

emotionally. Based on his own needs, Gary created blends such as Abundance, Believe, Highest Potential, Forgiveness, Inner Child and Trauma Life. During that 2016 convention, I had a number of profound experiences in the part of the expo dedicated to sampling every essential oil that Young Living produces. When I tested the Forgiveness blend, I started to think about who I would like to forgive, when all of a sudden, I broke down crying, right there, in the middle of the room. I thought, wow, these blends are powerful. After testing hundreds of the samples, I walked out floating. I was walking on a cloud with an immense smile on my face. I will call that, essential oil bliss!

As the earth provides everything that her children need, the plants have the properties to support our health and wellness. Young Living farms use only select seed, harvest with love and distill the highest quality therapeutic grade essential oils.

Question: So how do we fly upwards in our lives?
Answer: Start with Yoga and Essential Oils as a lifestyle. We can lift ourselves up physically, and therefore mentally, breathing in deeply the supporting aromas, flying through what I call: Bandha Life...

**breathe deeply
change your posture
change your attitude**

Journal for Yoga

What is your interpretation of Bandha? Practice engaging your core muscles throughout the day while breathing deeply, with good posture. Build the habit in your core. Write about how that makes you feel.

Full and Empty

It's such a delight to sit down with a good meal or drink and enjoy the flavors and company of others. Being full is half of the story. Yes, it's part of our survival as mammals to eat and drink and we do indulge profoundly, but according to yogic philosophy, we can also enjoy the feeling of being empty. I contemplated this deeply over many years after I learned about the Sanskrit word, kumbhaka* (koom-bah-kah), which means pot. I imagine kumbhaka as a clay pot from ancient India that held grain and water.

During our Pranayama exercises or breath control, we inhale and exhale deeply and rhythmically to bring the mind and therefore body into a state of peace, as when choppy water becomes still. Eventually, in our adult practice, we bring ourselves to retain the inhale for a series of seconds in what in Sanskrit is called the puraka kumbhaka (poo-rah-kah koom-bah-kah). We then exhale completely and hold the air out of our lungs for a series of seconds in what we call the rechaka kumbhaka (ray-cha-kah koom-bah-kah). It's the inhale and hold, then the exhale and hold.

The pot (lungs) can be held full of air or empty.

*Kumbhaka is the pause between an inhale and exhale. According to B.K.S. Iyengar, in his famous book: <u>Light on Yoga</u>, the "retention or holding the breath is a state where there is no inhalation or exhalation".

In the practice of yoga, we rejoice in emptiness equally to that of being full. On the whole, human beings relate 'food and nutrients' with love. And why not? Our first nurturing from Mother and Father were of warmth and sustenance. When we are fulfilled by our selves as adults and we let go of the need for Mother and Father to care for us, then we can freely explore our true needs. Every body has individual needs. I always say, "listen to your body". With this in mind, how do we relate to food, to emptiness?

As with the relationship between light and darkness, we see the qualities of being full as light and full of life, and empty as darkness, fear of letting go and fear of death. Ponder this for a while in your own life.

Contemplation Practice

• Imagine yourself surrounded by safety and abundance whether full or empty.

• Choose a Young Living essential oil that gives you happiness, add one drop to your palm, rub both palms together three times in a clockwise direction as in 'thrice round the mountain' setting your affirmation. With hands cupped over nose, breathe deeply for a while.

• Contemplate the topics of abundance and scarcity, light and darkness. Come to a place of peace.

• Understand that, as in Taoism, all opposites hold each other up in existence.

• Breathe deeply as the waves of goodness pour over you knowing that all things in nature wax and wane. So does the breath, the body, the stomach.

Start to understand that when you are hungry, it may be thirst. Bask in the inquiry of emptiness, drink water between meals and discover the hunger pain dissipate. Hey, emptiness is not so bad after all. I remember plenty of times when I was about to start my yoga Asanas with a hunger in the morning, but I drank a cup of water and the hunger washed away while I moved with the breath.

When I was about 10 years old, I went on a bicycle ride with my Dad down to Ocean Beach in San Francisco. During the ride along Golden Gate Park, I wanted to stop and get some food, but my Dad said, "drink water." Of course I didn't want to hear that, I wanted to go out to a restaurant and fill up with something yummy. In my adult life, I have reflected often on my father's wise words. With my own children, I have told them the same thing. Dad knew about the benefit of being empty and full and how to wait like a yogi. Now I add a drop of Peppermint Vitality™ to that water, to keep the yogi vibration high.

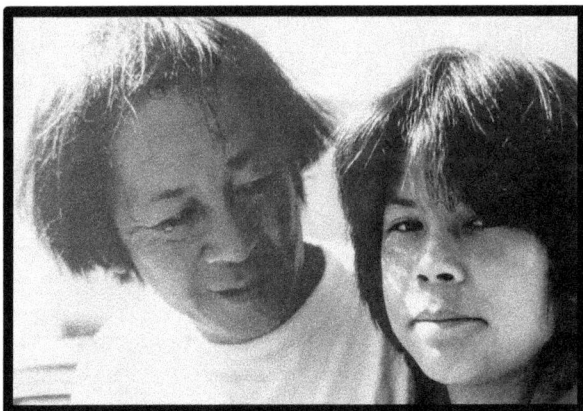

Journaling for Health

What do you think about being full versus empty? And what are some of your best practices of eating?

Yoga and Food

Each time you buy food, you vote in favor or against the earth and her children. We can take baby steps gaining collective exponential momentum towards a better world.

Consider taking one or more of the following steps:

1. Stop buying cow's milk, cheese, yogurt and butter (replace with delicious plant based alternatives, I love the almond-coconut blend for milk and coconut oil for butter)

2. Decide to stop or reduce your meat consumption (give our animal brothers and sisters your compassion)

3. Eat more organic greens (fruit and veggie smoothies and fresh pressed juices rock the alkaline lifestyle all day long), grow your own greens in the earth or planter boxes

Pretty soon, you start to feel uplifted, light and free. It takes time to let go of the mental, emotional and physical habits we have around the 'comfort foods' we have known from our childhoods (all cultures), but trust me, little by little, we can replace them with new healthy habits (delicious and simple ones, too). What's at stake? Our well being and that of our planet. A light lifestyle, a Bandha Life, is just around the corner when we decide to begin with baby steps.

Remember, according to the philosophy of Yoga, we can find comfort in emptiness as well as being full. Summer time is an excellent season to dwell in more liquid and emptiness without feeling suffering. Try smoothies with protein, teas and unsweetened lemonade to refresh. Give it a couple of months and that will bring you right into the Fall and Winter with a great new outlook (for the holiday season). Or jump right in during any season. The secret is to begin with one change, one alteration to our thought patterns and slowly take them on as our own. Over time, as with anything, the body and mind will accept the change as the norm.

Eternal blessings to you for your compassion for all beings.

One part liquid
One part solid
One part air
One part essential oils
~updated Ashtanga Yoga philosophy for meals

Journaling for Health

Where are some areas that you desire change in your eating and shopping habits?

KiDo Kids Yoga

We use Mindfulness and Yoga Philosophy together with YogaRhymes and Yoga Postures (Asanas) to enrich family's lives in homes and schools. Our very own KiDo Kids Yoga Preschool has been empowering little ones since 1999. Now in a digital format, anyone can enjoy our preschool program rich in stories, movement and activities.

YogaRhymes as the base of our KiDo Kids Yoga teacher trainings, have been going strong since 2006. Those catchy rhymes kids love to memorize and repeat with the poses, have traveled the four corners of the world. Our teachers are instructed not only how to teach and play yoga with all ages of children, but also how to incorporate sensory learning with Young Living essential oils.

We have trained teachers to lead classes with infants, toddlers and children through teens everywhere from Tokyo to Paris and Miami to Mexico. We are a Registered Children's Yoga School with Yoga Alliance offering online and in-person trainings.
On our website we also offer products, books and videos.

ESSENTIAL OILS

What makes Young Living the global leader in essential oils?
• seed to seal process
• therapeutic grade to support our health
• generous sharing rewards

On a visit to San Francisco's Yoga Journal Conference in 2009, I thought the main purpose was to connect with my Love Warrior Yoga crew: Duncan Wong and many other Epic Teachers. It wasn't until much later that I realized the most important part of that conference was a sweet smelling booth.
I had some downtime to browse through the fun offerings that were there and, like many others, I gravitated towards the booth that had the heavenly aromas misting up from mysterious little pools. It was my first exposure to Young Living and I quickly bought myself a kit of essential oils that came with a membership. Because I didn't understand the full possibility of health and wealth that were available through Young Living, when I used up my oils, I didn't take any action to order more.

With the encouragement of some of my close friends over the years, Young Living stayed in my life one way or another, but it wasn't until January of 2015 that I chose to build my oils business.
Young Living, the world leader in essential oils, has made

a huge difference in the quality of my family's health and spiritual well-being. It's not just the pure aroma, but the concentrated form of the plant that we benefit from. Mother Nature has all the answers for her children. Our roots to the Earth are as deep as the oldest trees.

All essential oils are not created equal.

Seed to Seal

Gary Young dedicated his life to creating Young Living. Over 20 years, he and his family reinvested their profits back into buying land and creating farms where Young Living continues to grow the highest quality plants that support all of our body systems.

The Seed to Seal promise focuses on the three primary elements of producing authentic essential oils of unmatched purity.

- Sourcing
- Science
- Standards

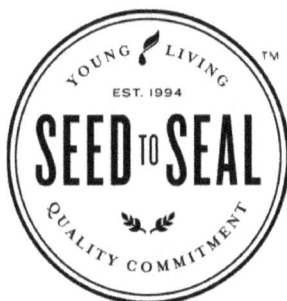

Sourcing

In this crazy world of seed manipulation, the source and quality of seed is crucial to the quality of product that we consume. The seeds selected to be grown on Young Living farms and Partner Farms come from plants that have been proven to produce the highest levels of bioactive compounds*. Therefore, the best quality essential oils are produced.

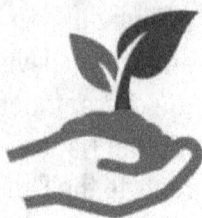

Can you imagine the thousands of acres of Young Living's sustainable farms? Gary Young always encouraged members to visit the farms and even help in the planting as an educational tool, but far before that, the preparation of the soil is what creates the greatest quality of the oil. We all know land degradation is a global problem, through deforestation and poor farming practices that deplete the soil. It's a refreshing stance when a company like Young Living cultivates the land with love, and the soil without chemicals (organic farming practices). Aromatic plants require a lot of nitrogen in order to produce oil. Good quality soil management is key in cultivating the enzymes that help the plant take up the minerals, vitamins and proteins.

*Bioactive compounds are extra nutritional constituents that occur in small quantities in foods and in concentrated quantities in essential oils.

Science

Gary Young studied the Art of Distillation in the 1990's with Henri Viaud, the Father of French Distillation, and Marcel Espieu, president of the Lavender Grower's Association in France for 20 years. Gary learned that there is a precise time to cut the plant, mature the plant (if required) and complete the amazing process of distillation* to produce the highest quality oils in the world.

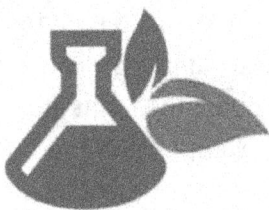

Why does Young Living have their own distilleries? Because the equipment is another key factor in the process. Other companies may only need the fragrance or flavoring molecules of the plant, but true

Young Living Therapeutic Grade™ (YLTG)

essential oils for topical and internal use are distinct to support our health, all of the molecules in the plant material must be distilled in the extraction chamber of the distillery. Every plant is distilled differently according to its active constituents (bioactive compounds or ingredients). Each essential oil must have the right proportions of constituents to meet the highest standard in the world that was set by Young Living.

*Distillation (by steam) is a separation process used to extract the essential oils from the plant material.

Why spend millions of dollars on lab equipment and lab technicians? For the same reason Young Living built the farms and distilleries, to analyze the chemical composition and the elements of the essential oils. This is how Young Living can guarantee consistent quality and purity.

The first order of business was to learn about how to analyze the oils, therefore Gary knew that he needed to return to France to study Gas Chromatography and Mass Spectrometry (GC-MS) analysis. GC provides a fingerprint of the essential oil by separating the components according to the differences in molecular volume. Basically, the essential oil is vaporized, then the rate of movement of each compound and its quantities are recorded. The MS further measures the presence and quantity of the exact constituents in each essential oil batch. This requires skill and experience. It was during his return to France that Gary met Dr. Herve Casabianca, the foremost authority in the world on Analytical Studies of Essentail Oils (the Chemistry of Essential Oils). **Dr. Casabianca eventually became the trainer for the technicians at the Young Living laboratory to teach them how to properly analyze the essential oils using the GC-MS analysis.**

Some studies are done in house and some are done in collaboration with other institutions such as Brigam Young University to document the quality. Associating with other Universities and Research Centers offers

backup or clarification if there is a question about the
testing of the quality of the essential oils.
Young Living essential oils exceed ISO and AFNOR
Standards**. From the extraction chambers in
distillation to the separators and finally to your bottle, the
essential oils will only ever touch steel or glass to control
the purity. For a complete education, as a member, just
like visiting a Young Living farm, you can participate in
the entire Seed to Seal process ending in filling the
bottles with essential oils, then putting on the caps and
labels.

Standards

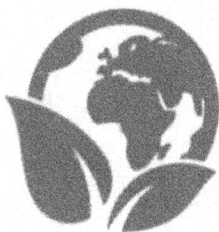

Commitment to the
highest quality of product
is tested through science,
commitment to the land is
practiced through sustainable farming,
making Young Living the leader in global standards.
From the selection of the seed and carefully cultivated
plants on the Young Living and partner farms to gentle,
steam distillation and scientific testing all sealed to be
mailed to you, the Seed to Seal promise is a complete
package to support your health and well being.

**The International Organization for Standardization (ISO),
founded in 1947, serve to safeguard consumers through a set
of standards and purity of essential oils.
**AFNOR (association française de normalisation) is a global
association governing standards based in France.

History of essential oils

Every culture throughout time have used plants as a support in family health. We can bring together the best of past and present technologies, by incorporating these ancient plant recipes into our modern lives. This aromatic liquid from shrubs, flowers, trees, roots, bushes and seeds is conveniently distilled and packaged for us by Young Living as a therapeutic grade essential oil. We can use it to support all of the body systems:

- aromatically
- topically
- internally

Our grandparents and their grandparents knew there is virtually no limit to the uses of plants in our lives and essential oils are the concentrated nutrients of plants. Because plants are linked to humans in this way, we can return to our birthright with the use of essential oils.

As early as 4500BCE, there are records describing aromatic substances for rituals and medical uses. Early forms of plant extracts have been documented in Egypt, Mesopotamia , Arabia, Crete, Greece and the Byzantine Empire. People of ancient times understood and used scented barks, resins, spices and aromatic vinegars in embalming, medicine, astrology, and temples. Egyptian masters of essential oils left hieroglyphs depicting oils and recipes such as at the Temple of Edfu where there was even a laboratory that used Frankincense and Myrrh.

Special vessels were carved out of alabaster to hold a

total of 350 liters of sacred essential oils in the tomb of King Tutankhamen. When the tomb was opened in 1922, only small amounts of the oils were left in the bottoms of the stone jars as thieves had stolen what was most important, essential oils.

The famous Ebers Papyrus from 1500BCE is one of the earliest medical records in history. This scroll of herbal knowledge is over 870 feet long (over 265 meters) with 877 prescriptions and recipes! It is currently kept at the library of the University of Leipzig, in Germany.

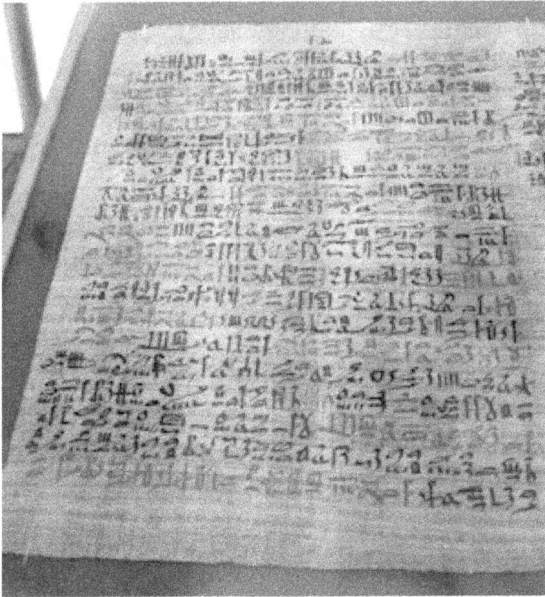

Essential Oils today

Aromatherapy gave way to total body support of essential oils with the mass popularity and boom in the 2000's. Most of us started our love of essential oils because of the attractive aroma, but with the Seed to Seal process of Young Living, the USFDA (United States Food and Drug Administration) approved the Vitality™ line of essential oils for ingestion! We can now add drops of our Young Living essential oils to our drinks, food and recipes. We can make our own supplements from 100% essential oils of plants by adding drops to clear vegetable capsules. Getting back to our roots, I say! So awesome.
As you've read in the Seed to Seal Promise, not all essential oils are created equal.

Here are some ideas for internal and external use:
• A glass of water with one drop of Vitality™ Peppermint (keep away from eyes, it is considered a hot oil)
• Powerhouse Frankincense massaged on the back of the neck to support wellness
• Thieves, the all time favorite for total support of the immune system, on the bottoms of the feet of adults and children
• Diffuse a few drops of relaxing Lavender at bedtime

Our ideas of how and why to use essential oils is expanding as the net is cast backward to ancient times. Our ancestors must be applauding the modern day 'oilers' for their dedication to what we may think of as a new fad, but according to history, are a timeless treasure. There are countless ways to better our lives with essential oils for adults, children and animals.

How 'Oilers Oil Up*' and you can too...

- Topically - apply 'neat' to skin or with a carrier oil
- Aromatically - one drop in palm, rub hands together, breathe in three or more times
- Internally - Vitality™ oils in a gelatin capsule, in your favorite drink or in cooking and baking

About the oils

These essential oils may be used 'Neat' which means directly on the skin full strength or diluted with a carrier oil. For children, we recommend diluting and using on the bottoms of their feet and on their spine.

If an essential oil gets in your eyes or other sensitive skin, you may use ample carrier oil (coconut oil, vegetable oil or YL's V-6 oil) in the affected area to reduce the burning sensation. Do not use water to reduce a burning sensation. Water enhances (or exacerbates) the warmth of an essential oil and a carrier oil reduces the burning sensation on skin or in eyes.

Do not use full strength oils on plastic surfaces or in plastic bottles as the essential oils do break down the plastics.

Only add essential oils to glass or stainless steel for drinking.

The Vitality™ oils have white labels indicating they are approved by the FDA for ingestion.

*Oilers are people who are super into essential oils. The term, "oil up", refers to applying oils internally and externally as health support.

Premium Starter Kit (PSK)

Includes: 12 essential oils + a diffuser and a wholesale membership. Your PSK is a key step into the Zing Living lifestyle. Combined with our best health practices and yoga, your new lifestyle is a snap. Learn a surprising variety of ways to use these oils everyday in every way for every family member (including infants, children and your furry family). Add drops of Vitality™ oils to your drinks, as supplements and with cooking.

1. Peppermint Vitality™ for energy support, digestion support and overall pick me up anytime, this is one of the Swiss Army knife oils that we never leave home without (along with Lavender).
Q: Is peppermint oil hot or is it cold?
A: Both, so keep away from eyes and sensitive skin! The menthol in peppermint oil has a cooling effect, but near the eyes or other sensitive skin, it has a burning sensation. It takes one pound of peppermint plant to make just one 15 milliliter bottle of this potent oil. Therefore, one drop goes a long way.
How to use Peppermint Vitality™ essential oil:
• add 1 drop to your water throughout the day for fresh breath, zesty wake up, to cool down and for digestive support (alternative to Digize™).
• apply to the back of your neck, shoulders or the soles of your feet to cool down on a hot day, with carrier oil opt
• add 1 drop to salad dressings, salsas, smoothies and baking for a compliment to sweet or savory recipes
• add 2+ drops to your diffuser for an uplifting ambiance
• find more ideas here: www.youngliving.com/blog

2. Lemon Vitality™ contains the essential oil from the peel of the lemon which contains limonene (an organic compound in the class of monoterpene), a potent support of the nervous system and emotions (think sunshine in a bottle). It offers a refreshing and clean aroma which helps to cleanse the body inside and out. And according to our grandparents, a great help in cleaning the surfaces of our homes (caution with plastic surfaces). Note: avoid going out in the sun after applying any citrus rind oil to the skin.

How to use Lemon Vitality™ essential oil:

- 2+ drops in the morning in your glass of water (with Peppermint Vitality™ optional)
- diffuse 2+ drops with water to uplift, support and focus
- 2+ drops in your night time moisturizer or skin cream
- 6+ drops in a spray bottle to refresh the air
- 3+ drops in your diffuser with purified water
- find more ideas here: www.youngliving.com/blog

3. Thieves Vitality™ is the famous Young Living immune system support blend from the essential oils of Clove, Lemon, Cinnamon, Eucalyptus and Rosemary. Because of its purifying, herbal qualities, it is used in the household cleaning and personal care products such as surface cleaner, dish soap, toothpaste and shampoo. The name comes from the story of four French thieves in the middle ages, who used a blend of clove, rosemary and other botanicals as a shield against the black death when they stole from the fallen victims during the bubonic plague.

With its spicy scent reminiscent of Winter holidays, this 'hot oil' should be handled with care as the cinnamon can have a burning feeling on the skin. Remember to use a carrier oil (such as coconut or vegetable oil), never water, to reduce a burning sensation on the skin.

How to use Thieves Vitality™ essential oil:

- boost your health daily 3+ drops in a vegetable capsule upgrade: Inner Defense supplement with Thieves
- rub 1+ drop on soles of feet, with carrier oil optional to support immune system in infants to adult
- 1 drop to your choice of heated milk + sweetener
- 2+ drops in dishwater or dishwasher to eliminate odor
- use in cooking and baking for extra spicy flavor boost
- 2+ drops in diffuser for a warm, welcoming scent

4. Citrus Fresh Vitality™ has the sunshine of

lemon with the benefit of friends. In this blend: Lemon invited Orange, Tangerine, Grapefruit, Mandarin Orange and Spearmint to the party! What a blast they all give. Remember the description of Lemon essential oil above, and that the organic compound, limonene, supports the nervous system, emotions and so much more? Imagine that potent boost times six, plus spearmint oil in the mix, which is gentler than peppermint, as a perfect compliment to this blend. You can also order Citrus Fresh Vitality™ to enjoy with your Summer beverages, all year round in your salsas and dressings, as well as in your cooking and baked goods. Note: avoid going out in the sun after applying any citrus rind oil to the skin.

How to use Citrus Fresh™ essential oil:

- diffuse 4+ drops to neutralize odors in all your rooms
- apply 2+ drops to a cotton ball for call vent or home
- 2+ drops in your favorite drink or over fresh fruit salad

5. Digize Vitality™ will become your go to oil for home and travel stomach and digestive discomfort. This blend of Tarragon, Ginger, Peppermint, Juniper, Fennel, Lemongrass, Anise, and Patchouli sound like a gourmet salad of herbs from a five star restaurant, and as essential oils, they aid in digestion and offer a fresh-tasting follow-up to any meal.

How to use Digize Vitality™ essential oil:

- 2+ drops in water or in a gelatin capsule to support digestion anytime you feel digestive discomfort
- 1+ drop in water to alleviate stomach discomfort when traveling (like riding in the backseat on winding roads)
- diffuse in the car when driving for above discomfort

6. Raven™ is another oil to keep on hand during the cold, Winter months together with Thieves. In the language of the Malagasy People of Madagascar, the famous Ravintsara means: the tree with good leaves. Ravintsara, together with Lemon, Wintergreen, Peppermint and Eucalyptus form the Raven blend of essential oils that supports the lungs and healthy respiratory function.

How to use Raven™ essential oil:

- apply to neck, chest and upper back 'neat' or with a carrier oil to support lungs and respiratory function
- rub 2+ drops on the soles of your feet before sleep
- add 2+ drops to diffuser for a fresh, crisp atmosphere

7. Valor™ brings out your inner Hero! Blending the essential oils of three powerful trees with a gentle flower: Black Spruce, Rosewood, Frankincense and Blue Tansy. This special blend is used to balance and align our energy as the first oil in a popular version of Gary Young's Neuro

Auricular Technique (NAT). Give your friends and family the famous NAT oils experience with 1. Valor (the balancer), then 2. Frankincense (the brain support), next 3. Peppermint (or Panaway, the deep driver), and finally, 4. Copaiba (the amplifier). Simply add a rollerball fitment to each bottle, then apply the oils to the brainstem (occipital ridge at the base of the skull where the indentation is felt) in a circular motion. Extend the experience by rolling each oil up and down either side of the vertebae on the back of the neck from the C5 vertebrae to the brainstem and back down again.

How to use Valor essential oil:
- 1 drop on palm, rub palms, cup over nose, breathe 3 x
- find more ideas here: www.youngliving.com/blog

8. Panaway™ is soothing and stimulating with a combination of Wintergreen, Helichrysum, Clove and Peppermint essential oils. Open this little bottle and let the genie out with the magical, minty aroma. Let the cares of the world float away when Panaway is on your team. Whether you rub it on a tender muscle to soothe or on the back of your neck and temple to stimulate. Enjoy the sensation of being relaxed and aware at the same time.

How to use Panaway™ essential oil:
- rub 1+ drop with carrier oil to massage muscles after your workout or whenever your muscles feel tender
- 1 drop in palm, dab to apply to temples at hairline keep far back from eyes as this blend has 'hot' oils
- with rollerball fitment, apply to the back of your neck
- find more ideas here: www.youngliving.com/blog

9. Lavender is a classic aroma that actually has dozens of varieties. The variety called Lavandula Angustifolia was chosen by Young Living for it's health supporting benefits for use with their Lavender essential oil and Lavender Vitality™ essential oil. The choice of this variety is a key distinction in the quality of the oil, for topical, aromatic and internal uses. Right there in the Simiane Valley of charming Provence, France is the Simiane-la-Rotonde Lavender Farm owned by Young Living. We can say, this is the area where it all started, where Gary Young learned the art of distillation from the old masters who eventually, with trusting love, gifted him the coveted lavender seed. The rest is history.

Lavender from Young Living, like Thieves™ is used in a multitude of products from personal care to baby products to all of the essential oil blends.

Lavender Vitality™ essential oil, which is labeled for consumption, is beneficial for not only deep relaxation, and health support, but can also be used to enhance your favorite cold beverages, in savory dishes and baking adventures.

How to use Lavender essential oil:

- add 4+ drops each of Lavender, Lemon and Peppermint in a vegetable capsule for seasonal discomfort and general health support

- diffuse 2+ drops at bedtime to promote calm and relaxation anytime, but especially for a restful night

- rub 2+ drops on sensitive skin areas with carrier oil

- add 3+ drops in a spray bottle with purified water to freshen any room with a floral, clean aroma

10. Frankincense historically has been sought after to elevate the human spiritual existence. For the past 5000 years, Frankincense resin has been distilled in the capital of Oman called Muscat. Young Living is the only company who has permission to harvest and export from these sacred trees. Frankincense Vitality™ also may support the brain and normal cell health taken as a supplement.

How to use Frankincense essential oil:

- 1 drop in palm, rub together, cup nose, breathe aroma
- 1+ drop applied to skin around eyes to reduce the appearance of fine lines while supporting vision
- diffuse 3+ drops when practicing all branches of yoga

11. Stress Away™ is a surprisingly complex blend that just smells like cake (that's what kid's say). Grownups also love aromas that smell like food. Many use this blend of Vanilla extract with the essential oils of Lime, Lavender, Copaiba, Cedarwood and Ocotea as perfume on the neck and wrists. The aroma is calming, comforting, and sweet. Melt away from stress by simply inhaling this blend anytime. Stress Away also helps alleviate occasional nervous irritability and uplift the senses.

How to use Stress Away™ essential oil:

- add roller fitment and apply to neck and wrists for anytime boost of smiles for all ages: child, teen, adult
- diffuse 2+ drops in water for a welcoming room
- 1 drop in palm, rub together, cup nose, breathe aroma to promote relaxation and a calm
- add 1+ drop to a cottonball for car vent to freshen air

12. Peace & Calming™ is just what you need during busy days and before bed for a restful night. Imagine the light citrus scents of Tangerine and Orange, the floral aromas of Ylang Ylang and Blue Tansy, grounded with the earthy grit of long lasting patchouli. The highs and lows together in a timeless blend.
How to use Peace & Calming™ essential oil:
• diffuse 3+ drops for day or night relaxation
• massage 2+ drops on bottoms of feet neat or diluted
• 1 drop in palm, rub together, cup nose, breathe aroma
• add 2+ drops in bath for aromatic relaxation
• add 1+ drop to a cottonball for car vent to freshen air

Warnings and precautions: Keep essential oils out of reach of children. These products are not intended to diagnose, treat, cure or prevent any disease. Essential oils for external use, except the Vitality™ product line. Avoid eyes and mucous membranes. If you are pregnant, nursing, taking medication, or have a medical condition, consult a health professional prior to use. This book has not been evaluated by the Food and Drug Administration nor by Young Living essential oils, although, all facts have been taken from the Young Living books, sources and websites in honor of Gary Young.

Journaling for Essential Oils

When you open each bottle of oil, what are your first reactions? Over time, depending upon our state of mind, health, and all, our reaction to an oil may change.

Fascinating Science Facts about essential oil constituents:
• The first smells in a blend are the monoterpenes or top notes, which have smaller molecules. They reach across and fill a room quickly, but also evaporate faster (such as Peppermint essential oil).
• The subsequent smells, are called middle and base notes which come from the sesquiterpenes that move more slowly, tend to be a thicker consistency and stay on surfaces longer (such as Sandalwood essential oil).

Love it, Share it

Become a true 'Oiler' and carry these 12 everyday oils with you in a handy traveling oils case that fits right in your bag, briefcase or backpack. Your essential oils will be your allies in a tough world. You know you can already handle life's situations, and now you can do it all with calm and confidence. When we love a product so much, we usually want to share with others. Young Living has a generous Compensation Plan for those who share and enroll others with a Premium Starter Kit. This is the way Young Living works, as a direct marketing business, paying its distributors for word-of-mouth networking. You can dabble in sharing as a fun social business and earn extra money in the process, or stick with only personal use as a Preferred Customer.

1 Purchase a Premium Starter Kit for **Personal Use**, receive your 12 therapeutic grade essential oils, diffuser, Member Number, 24% discount, Virtual Office online, and Preferred Customer status Optional custom monthly box: Essential Rewards Millions of members are Preferred Customers

2 Become a **Business Builder** by enrolling another, start as a Distributor, then build your YL business, Young Living sends $50 for enrolling each person Top Compensation Plan + Rockin Global Conventions

If you don't have a sponsor or enroller, you are welcome to join our Zing Living Team with Member # 2391868. www.myYL.com/KiDoKids www.KiDoKidsYoga.com

YOUNG LIVING 2017 WORLDWIDE INCOME DISCLOSURE STATEMENT

WORLDWIDE INCOME STATISTICS FOR JANUARY-DECEMBER 2017

WHAT ARE MY EARNING OPPORTUNITIES? This document provides statistical, fiscal data about the average member income and information about achieving various ranks.

YOUNG LIVING MEMBER RANK	PERCENTAGE OF ALL BUSINESS BUILDERS[1]	MONTHLY INCOME[2]				ANNUALIZED AVERAGE INCOME[3]	AVERAGE MONTHS TO ACHIEVE RANK[4]		
		Lowest	Highest	Median	Average		Low	Average	High
DISTRIBUTOR	33.3%	$0	$725	$15	$26	$312	N/A	N/A	N/A
STAR	41.02%	$0	$932	$58	$75	$906	1	12	267
SENIOR STAR	15.66%	$2	$5,531	$193	$235	$2,819	1	19	255
EXECUTIVE	6.62%	$34	$13,210	$425	$502	$6,028	1	25	254
SILVER	2.55%	$229	$29,248	$1,698	$2,088	$25,059	1	32	252
GOLD	0.57%	$1,506	$48,630	$4,541	$5,666	$67,995	2	49	263
PLATINUM	0.18%	$4,375	$90,275	$11,057	$13,872	$166,468	5	58	243
DIAMOND	0.07%	$6,256	$163,387	$27,972	$35,348	$424,178	7	70	251
CROWN DIAMOND	0.01%	$28,492	$231,397	$53,589	$64,477	$773,724	16	85	258
ROYAL CROWN DIAMOND	0.02%	$50,770	$326,334	$132,826	$144,551	$1,734,606	17	97	230

[1] Because a member's rank may change during the year, these percentages are not based on individual member ranks throughout the entire year but are based on the average distribution of member ranks during the entire year. Business Builders are members who have personally enrolled at least one other person and does not include Preferred Customers.

[2] Because a member's rank may change during the year, these incomes are not not based on individual member incomes throughout the entire year but are based on earnings of all members qualifying for each rank during any month throughout the year.

[3] This is calculated by multiplying the average monthly incomes by 12. These incomes include income earned from January 1, 2017, through December 31, 2017, but which was paid between February 2017 and January 2018.

[4] These statistics include all historical ranking data for each rank and thus are not limited to people who achieved these ranks in 2017. Members who do not make at least one product purchase in the previous 12 months are considered inactive.

The income statistics in this statement are for incomes earned by all worldwide active Business Builder members in 2017. An "active Business Builder" member is a member who made at least one product purchase in the previous 12 months and has personally enrolled at least one person during the lifetime of the member account. The average annualized income of the member account was $684, and the median Business Builder members in this time was $3,321; and the median annualized income was $684.

Note that the compensation paid to members summarized in this disclosure does not include expenses incurred by members in the operation or promotion of their business, which can vary widely and might include advertising or promotional expenses, product samples, training, rent, travel, telephone and internet costs, and miscellaneous expenses. The earnings of the members in this chart are not necessarily representative of the income, if any, that a Young Living member can or will earn through the Young Living Compensation Plan. These figures should not be considered as guarantees or projections of your actual earnings or profits. Young Living does not guarantee any income or rank success.

61

notes

Essential Rewards

Just one drop is a lot, but when your essential oils run out, order more with an abundant attitude! And make sure to check out all the amazing products in the product guide and on the website:

• single oils, blends, home care, bath & body care
• baby products, animal care,
• nutrition, fitness, weight management supplement recommendations: Ningxia Red™, Inner Defense™, Multigreen™, Agilese™, Life 9™ Progessence Plus™ for women & Shutran™ for men

After ordering your Premium Starter Kit, make sure to choose your custom monthly box as an autoship order through the Essential Rewards Program by going to:

www.YoungLiving.com then signing in with your...

Member Number_____

Password _____

Find the Virtual Office, then Essential Rewards. Make sure to take advantage of YL Go to receive free two day shipping every month (see details in the Virtual Office). While you're in your Virtual Office, have a look around. There you will find everything you need including your Dashboard (Getting Started tab) and Member Resources.

Use your Essential Oils pocket Reference from Life Science as an encyclopedia of support in book form or as an app on smart phones.

Here's to your Wellness, Purpose & Abundance!

ACTION

A Health, Yoga and Young Living Essential Oil lifestyle combined with Action are the tools that have worked to manifest my dream life. I thought, if I can do it, then why can't others duplicate what I have created?

Boom! Enter Zing Living.

If I manifested greatness while giving back to my community, then what's stopping anyone from getting there? Simply, it could be a lack of motivation or a lack of action. We all get stuck sometimes, now we can use this book over and over to keep moving forward. Yes, I keep going back to read my own book, to remember again and again what has worked.

In Zing Living, Action refers to many things:
• consistently taking action
• personal growth
• tools to keep in action

Without taking action, the spark of your dreams may fizzle out. On the other hand, moving forward with completing your daily tasks (large and minute) will create the momentum that lead to your goals. We all know this, but removing the obstacles (both mental and physical) that keep us in a fog each day, each breath, is the key.

Removing Obstacles

How to remove those obstacles?
First, identify what is stopping you. Is it a lack of energy, physical limitations or confusion? Do you just feel defeated and unsure of where to begin?
Have you forgotten your dreams?

What stops you from taking actions?

List the top 5 reasons you think you pause or stop instead of taking the actions you know will forward you in your life.

1

2

3

4

5

Journaling for Action

Looking at the 5 reasons you listed, when in your life have you seen that pattern before? When was the first time you remember starting this pattern?

Now powerfully choose to move forward with Action.

Do you believe that action comes from motivation? The greatest accomplishments in this world all came from the seed of a thought that grew with strong emotion into action. If motivation comes from emotion, then how do we stir up that emotion?

thought --> emotion --> motivation --> action

Whether you are bursting with ideas and motivation, or feel it's been too long (or never) since you felt that natural high with ideas popping and the motivation to get it all complete.

Right now you hold in your hands the possibility of greatness. Breathe deeply and give that thought a chance.

How do we stir up our best thoughts and emotions? Do you allow yourself to get excited over ideas and possibilities?
Let's take a stroll through what lights us up.

Find a comfortable, quiet place to sit or lie down. Close your eyes and focus on your breath. Notice what you are feeling in your body. Go down through the layers of relaxation allowing each moment to be what it is (not judging yourself). When your body has acclimated to the position, you may feel a floating sensation. Stay there. Do not let sleep enter yet, but instead, invite yourself to stay in that relaxation and engage in questions. Give yourself permission to be guided to receive the messages of your highest dreams. Ask yourself, "What lights me up? What is my highest potential? How can I best serve myself and others? Stay in that place of inquiry and notice the answers that come through. When you are ready, return to this book and on the next few pages write down your insights. When you have finished, if you want to take a nap, my Dad said it was a good idea...

Once when my Dad was teaching me how to use the I Ching* (ee-cheeng) or Book of Changes, which is an ancient Chinese process of divination, I said, "Why do I get sleepy after I toss the coins?" In his infinite wisdom he replied, "Your conscious and subconscious brain want to unite and they can do so during sleep." He told me this one time, and I will never forget. Thanks Dad! There are many ways to remove obstacles and gain clarity opening channels for motivation and action.

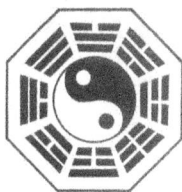

*The I Ching uses three coins or a bundle of sticks that are tossed thoughtfully to the ground with a question in mind. The result of how the coins or sticks fall are used to make calculations with a manual for a series of solid and broken lines which result in poetic readings as divinations. According to my Dad, Victor Wong, this is not fortune telling, it is tapping into the infinite wisdom connecting our movements (such as tossing coins) to a higher source.

Journaling for Action

What lights you up?
Write the details of what lights you up.

How can I best serve myself and others?

In this chapter, I'm going to outline a great path to clearing and cleaning the mental and physical obstacles that may be standing in your way of achieving your best life. Being organized in your home and workplace are key to staying focused with your goals. I believe that working on the physical, leads to the mental. Let's start with the challenging, yet refreshing act of clearing your spaces.

On a scale of 1 to 10, circle the number which represents your level of organization in life (1 being the least organized and 10 being the most organized). If negative thoughts come up for you in this process, allow those thoughts to pass by and not attach to them. Keep your spirit light and if you get too heavy, reach out to someone close to you to talk. The key here is to identify obstacles, remove them and keep moving forward in the direction you choose. Keep in Action.

1 2 3 4 5 6 7 8 9 10

---

challenge:

- don't attach to negative thoughts
- keep it light and trust the process
- clearing your spaces will inevitably clear your mind

Here are some examples of obstacles:
- emotional obstacles (can't let go of things)
- physical obstacles (where to put everything)
- lack of energy (you just feel heavy with the weight)

Journaling for Action

In the past, what have been the major obstacles that stop you from clearing your spaces?

Uncluttered Spaces

Imagine for a moment, your home and work space completely clear and clean. Surfaces are gleaming in the sunlight, the curtains are wafting in the cool, sweet smelling breeze, and you can hear the sound of children playing and laughing in the distance.

Clearing and cleaning your home and work space is such a personal process. Each article may have a memory attached to it, an emotional charge on us. Whereas piles of paperwork, mail, magazines and newspapers may have none. Commit to going through the cluttered areas with a warrior's perseverance. For those delicate pieces, lovingly dust them off, wrap them and place them gently in boxes to be stored. Get a storage unit if you don't have an on site area where boxes can be stored. Get rid of the extra things which are weighing you down. The process of decluttering your spaces is very healing, likened to an inner and outer cleansing.

When I clean my spaces, I notice I smile and laugh more. My attitude changes.

Keep your goal in mind:
"to clear and clean until you have
an uncluttered home and work space"
It may take a series of hours, days, weeks or months (or in my case, years), but I give you permission to not give up. You will thank me later, now get to it!

Journaling for Action

List here what rooms in your home and work space are cluttered and what is cluttering them.

Suggested items for Organizing

- Trays and a sheet
- Boxes or Tubs (free or purchased)
- Files for filing system
- File sized boxes or filing cabinet
- Off site storage unit

Strategy for Uncluttering Spaces

- Look at your list of rooms and spaces to be uncluttered
- Allot times in your week dedicated to only this task
- Choose one room to attack
- Take each room in sections or by category of items (i.e. clothing, paper, shelf, table, etc)
- Gather loose items onto a tray, then sort into piles, put away piles after sorting is done
- Spread a sheet out on the floor for large amounts of paperwork or other loose items, sort, put away
- Sorting can be fun to do while listening to the radio, an audio book or watching TV
- Methodically go through each room on your mental or written list
- Be patient with the process, work consistently, don't give up half way through
- Emotional attachment to physical things is common, letting go gives us a profound sense of freedom
- Work steadily everyday (or set forth your schedule and stick to it) to complete the tasks

Digging a little deeper...

Just before I began to write this section, I went through a crazy thorough clearing and organizing of my spaces. Some paperwork I had pushed to the side for years, finally emerged and went to recycling. I made boxes of labeled files and projects to be accessed with ease for later. I would dump bags of stuff onto sheets and trays, then watch episodes of my current favorite show while organizing. I began to feel more light and free, especially seeing the corners of rooms, shelves and floor space free up. I was unconsciously living the process while writing about it, what a trip! My younger son was at Summer Camp in Oregon, so after organizing all of my spaces, I decided to keep the momentum flowing and jumped in to cleaning his room. Because he was getting into his teens, I knew there were lots of childhood mementos in his room that a young man wouldn't want there anymore. They were just taking up space. I'm a big kid who loves to collect toys, just like my Dad was, so I dove in and enjoyed walking down memory lane hour after hour sorting toys that went back to my older son's collections from 15 years before. I realized at a certain point while I was lovingly placing the miniature racing cars in their box that I wouldn't be unpacking these again until the next generation of little ones are born. Sweet and Sad at the same time. I hope you enjoy your process as much as I did.

The process has begun...keep up the clearing of the physical as an ongoing habit (we all know how 'things' accumulate every week). Use that habit as a weekly ritual with enjoyment. Celebrate your successes and note the process both mental and physical of clearing and cleaning your spaces. The lighter we are, the more power we have to attract what 'lights us up'...and the energy to best serve ourselves and others.

Journaling for Action

Write about your successes in clearing and organizing.

Clearing the physical spaces was half the work. In our commitment to ourselves, to what is possible, we must also toss out the old stories we are holding onto. This is easier said than done, as we feel the old stories '*are* who we are'.

Let's look at what I'm talking about here...

What are your secret dreams? The ones so big they scare you. Let's reframe that thinking. The main reason we connect fear with achieving our dreams is that we don't believe we are worthy. The judgement of being worthy or unworthy was bestowed upon us as children and young people. Whether spoken or absorbed through the environment, we have written entire volumes of stories in our heads about what we do or do not deserve. These books, we carry as reality, become so blessedly heavy, we become weighted down by the very creation we ourselves conjured as children. I say, it's time to Wake Up from that story, from that loop of negative thoughts. From those patterns that do not serve us.

Are you ready to step outside of your old paradigm and set your wild self free?

Just shed the old ways like a cat sheds their fur in the Summer. It's naturally healthy. It's life giving. The people around us will notice a difference and that is wonderful.   #scarybigiscool

Stepping into the unknown...

Once, I had the opportunity to recreate my life out of a visit to Guatemala. Spirit granted me a boon that I had prayed for during the previous years in San Francisco while I was attending design school and swimming in the underground culture of dance and fashion. During this visit, I found the most amazing native town of Kak'chikeles in a place called Sololá along the edge of Lake Atitlán. Lifetimes away from the busy city I was born in, I met an enchanting young man. In fact, he was so enchanting that I decided to stay. This boon granted to me had beautiful black hair and cinnamon skin with a gentle voice and matching kindness. His family became my family; I happily married into the rich, Mayan culture. I recreated my life in an instant and have never looked back. Throughout our life together, we have broken out of story after story from our respective childhoods. From our first adobe brick home built by a local cousin and filled with our own hand made furniture in Sololá to our flower and herb garden home in Northern California were we now reside over 25 years later, we have struggled with our individual insecurities. The story of not being worthy, of not being good enough, of being too shy to speak our truths, is so deeply ingrained, but the love we have for each other and for ourselves has triumphed again and again. We certainly are not the same people we were in 1992 when we first met, but our essences have flourished and our dreams continue to grow together.

How can we shed the old ways? It's rather simple. It has been said that it takes at least two weeks to create a habit. If you can identify the small victories, the clear decisions, the improvements, then you can find patience with this process.

Remember, your dream life is worth it!

When we repeatedly replace the old stories with new ones and take consecutive actions towards those dreams and goals, then we can recreate our lives again and again. We can impress and inspire ourselves and those around us to keep on track and keep building dreams and visions together. When we convince our brains that the new story we create is real, we naturally live into that new reality.

When we watch a movie or show with top notch acting, we fall into the story as if we are there (thank you beautiful actors). It has also been said that our minds cannot distinguish between the screen and reality. We cease to see what is around us and begin to feel what the movie or show feeds us, be it love or violence, passion or intrigue. Our hearts race when we see the edge of the precipice or the car speeding down the road, equally we melt when the lovers kiss.

Let's create our own epic tale to live in to, to fall in love with. And it all begins with a decision to set our **wild selves free**. Our most secret dreams, the ones so big they scare us, are within our reach.

I say, "That which we can envision powerfully is bound toward us." Life has no guarantees, but we choose to see our success ahead of us.

old story --> new story --> goals --> action

Here are four powerful steps to work toward what lights you up:

• Rewrite new stories that light you up

• Create your overall goals

• Break the overall goals into micro steps

• Make vision boards

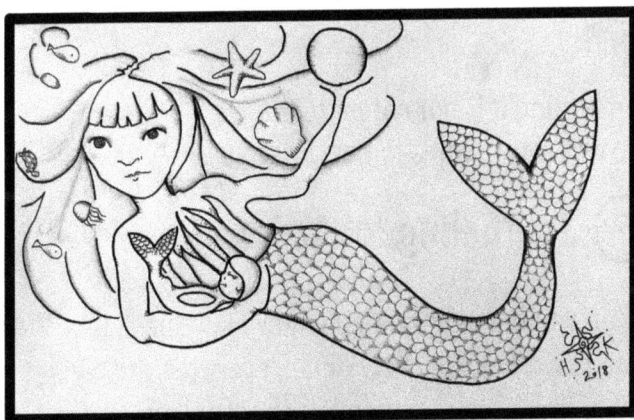

Always keep swimming towards your goals.

Rewrite a New Story

Plan a quiet time alone, without interruption, to imagine, to remember and to be open to what dreams may flow through. Make sure to silence your phone and computer. Relax and breathe deeply. See yourself as safe and happy, with everything you need. Say to yourself, if I could have anything I desired, (without greed or negative intentions) then what would it be?

Dive deeply in to this vision

Feel your spirit soar with lightness, understand your value in the world. Know that you are worthy of greatness and can now help others find their self worth. Note the way it feels and how everything looks, the way this new world smells and appeals to you. If emotions emerge, let them flow forth to make space for your new story.

Remember, it is our nature to thrive.
The very earth wants to give this to us.

Journaling for Action

When you have completed your vision quest, take the time to write down every detail, every texture, every smell, every color (on another sheet or your journal).

Create Your Goals

Creating your goals are as easy as extracting the main themes of your new story, your new dream that you draw power from. Write those main themes on large pieces of paper as overall goals to be achieved. Post those words with matching images around your home.
Really dig in to the idea of **your self worth** and be stubborn about it.

Power words to post where you can see them daily: (though you may not feel or believe your statements, say them out loud with emotion daily, throughout the day)

My life is worthy

I am deeply in love with myself

I am valuable in my community

Write three phrases that begin with 'I am...', then rewrite them on a large sheet of paper in bold to be tacked on your wall where you will see them everyday (throughout the day).

1. I am

2. I am

3. I am

Don't give up easily, even when the odds are against you. There is no doubt in my mind about the extreme value each individual can have on their communities. Be it a child, a young person, an adult or an animal, the positive actions we take DO impact others. Many indigenous cultures believe we are the connection between sky and earth, a potent conductor of all that is possible.

Remember your dream often and repeat those positive words aloud every day, speaking the power of the new story into reality.

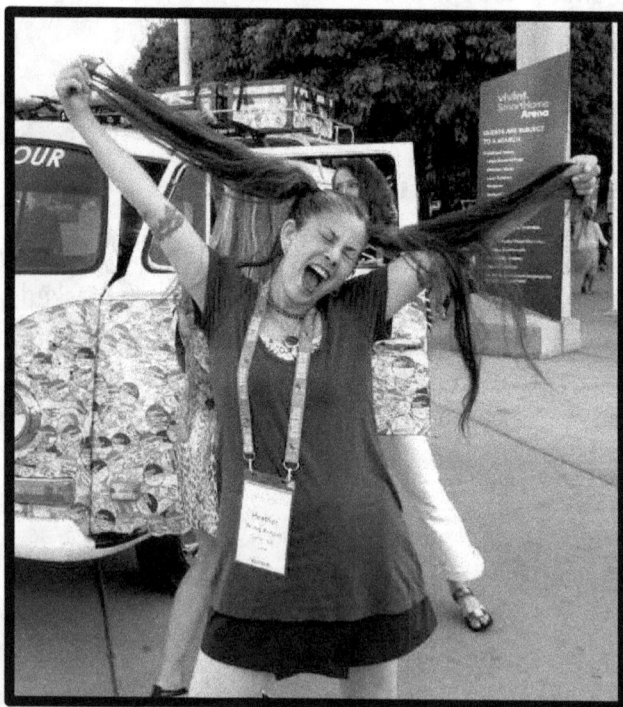

2016 International Grand Convention SLC, Utah

We create the life that nurtures us, that in turn we can help others.

"Our deepest fear is not that we are inadequate. Our deepest fear is that we are powerful beyond measure. It is our light, not our darkness that most frightens us. We ask ourselves, 'Who am I to be brilliant, gorgeous, talented, fabulous?' Actually, who are you not to be? You are a child of God. Your playing small does not serve the world. There is nothing enlightened about shrinking so that other people won't feel insecure around you. We are all meant to shine, as children do. We were born to make manifest the glory of God that is within us. It's not just in some of us; it's in everyone. And as we let our own light shine, we unconsciously give other people permission to do the same. As we are liberated from our own fear, our presence automatically liberates others."

~Marianne Williamson

And another beautiful, inspiring quote that makes a person second guess the purpose of fear.

"Perhaps all the dragons in our lives are princesses who are only waiting to see us act, just once, with beauty and courage. Perhaps everything that frightens us is, in its deepest essence, something helpless that wants our love."

~Rainer Maria Rilke

Micro Steps

Create micro steps of your goals from your new story. Take the time to really think through how small tasks can work toward your dreams, even if that means years down the road. This is the part that takes immense patience, but as you follow through with these powerful steps to recreate your story, you will begin to feel a new reality is setting into place. Be open to miracles and know that you are consciously and subconsciously taking the correct actions to fulfill your dreams. Remember, it's the little things that add up to greatness. Everyday, not giving up. Everyday, taking micro actions, micro steps toward your larger goals. No matter how boring it feels, keep your strong vision in mind.

Journaling for Action

The micro steps I will take are:

Though it scared the pants off me...

I pursued my dream of being a yoga teacher. About 1998, I asked my brother, Duncan, to hold the vision of me as a teacher because I couldn't bare to think of myself in front of people, teaching. The fear was so deep, it made me shudder, and yet, I was driven toward it. I had done many things in my full life. I had danced, traveled the world, designed clothing, became a Mama, but the fear continued to eat away at me. I was slowly unwinding the old stories and replacing them with becoming a Fearless Warrior. In 2005, I took my first yoga teacher training, in Yogic Arts, and repeated the same course multiple times, year after year with my brother. I began to create KiDo Kids Yoga and traveled to Japan with it, where Duncan resided. Every time I traveled, I was filled with fear, but I always showed up with greatness. I brought my younger son with me every year, he watched me go through my rituals of fear and breakthrough to bravery. The experience completely changed both of our lives. He was the only one who saw it, he and my family, but my students only saw the bravery in me and that was correct. I pushed through what felt like lifetimes of deep seeded fear and eight years later, I arrived to Japan, with my son, who had now grown taller than me, feeling relaxed and knowing how to communicate in Japanese and find my way around the country by train. Eventually, and without noticing, I became a master teacher on three continents and melted away my fear.
This girl dominated fear and you can, too.

As a promise to yourself, keeping the life of your dreams always within your thoughts, you can sign the letter on the next page and print it.
Sign it with passion! Smile, you are on your way.

Your daily homework is to form the new habit of loving yourself, knowing your worth, and knowing that your gifts can help others.

When you have moments of negativity, ask yourself:
- How is my breathing pattern?
- Have I been keeping moving (exercise)?
- What have I been consuming?
- What have I been drinking?
- Am I keeping in touch with friends or a coach to talk and keep open in the world?
- Am I using my Young Living essential oils to raise my frequency and support my health?

Now breathe deeply reciting love for yourself, go for a walk, do some yoga stretches or other exercise, eat and drink something healthy (with a friend if possible), and oil up for health! Advice from my Dad about moments of negativity, "Always do your best to dissolve the negativity [be it alone or with others] with a good attitude in the moment. Later, you will be pleased about how you acted, versus allowing the negativity to consume you and bitterly regretting it later".

Promise to yourself (sign with passion):

Dear New Story,
I promise to love you and to nurture our relationship which is growing. Even though I know the old stories will try to tear me away from you (they will try again and again in clever ways to get me back) I will sweep them away just like the dirt I sweep out of my home. I see clearly that the old stories are not life giving and certainly not loving me. And you, dear possibility, dear New Story, will bring my dreams to fruition.
I will repeat everyday for you...

I am worthy of big dreams

I am brave when I feel fear

I step back from the negative

I breathe deeply and love myself

I let go

I forgive

I am _____

I have _____

With All My Heart,

signed _____

date _____

Vision Boards

Vision Boards are for manifesting.

The final point with these four powerful steps to letting go of the old story and welcoming the new is the creation of your custom Vision Board, also known as a Dream Board. This is a tool to bring a sharp focus to your life, as Olympic athletes and countless others have done.

The higher purpose here is to keep an image in view and believe that is possible to attain. I like the old saying, "Fake it 'til you Make it". More eloquently put by Thoreau, "Go confidently in the direction of your dreams. Live the life you have imagined." The Vision Board is the life you have imagined.

A Vision Board can be a simple statement written and accompanied by pictures you have chosen or a collage of many images and words. It can be small or large, but no matter the size, to get the results...

keep it where you will see it daily

I encourage you to make many vision boards and post them all around your home and office. Keep your vision boards current by updating or creating new versions often as your dreams will evolve.

You can buy a bulletin board, poster board, tag board paper or even a spiral bound drawing paper pad to make your Vision Board. It can be made by adding images and matching text that you print, draw or rip out of old magazines.

Before you begin the process, I recommend getting into a very grounded place and focusing on your goals.

Detailed instructions for making your Vision Board:
to your...

• bulletin board made of cork or

• simple sheet of colored cardboard or

• any sheet of paper

Add images and words printed out, drawn or cut out from a magazine.

• Use push pins, sewing pins, tape or glue to attach pictures and words

• Choose images and words based on your dreams and visions

• Use images that call you to action, that light you up.

• Remember to keep your vision board clear of clutter, current and full of inspiration

With a clear picture of your long term vision you can master your path. Scientists say, we are imprinting the image on our minds and creating a physical pathway which becomes a habit (be it thought or action).
Find more vision board inspiration on our website and across the internet.

Spirit Secretary

What if you could empty out your heavy thoughts, your long to do lists to a higher place.
What if you could have your own personal secretary.

Breathe Deeply, know
that you can.
Right here,
right now.

Spirit Secretary is
always there for you...
keeping you Organized,
                    Sorted and
                        Perfectly Timed.

Let your thoughts float up to the sky.
You will be reminded when the time is correct.
Look out for the clever ways Spirit reminds you to get something done. Perhaps a license plate, a sign, a note catching your attention, the radio, words on a friend's lips, your own mind catching the message...all just in time to get that task done by deadline.

We still use our paper organizers, but the body is relaxed and full of faith...all the while being Organized, Sorted and Perfectly Timed on all levels.

Let me explain...

After a KiDo Kids Yoga tour to Japan in 2011, I was lying in bed awake, jet lagged 2:00am, thinking about the long to do list I had ahead of me. The many tasks, promises to be kept to my new students and work at home were packed into my brain. It occurred to me that I needed a secretary and at that time, the possibility of having one seemed highly unlikely. Next thought: what if I could alleviate my dear, packed brain by extracting the tasks one by one and placing them into the space above my head, neatly ordered, side by side, for my Spirit to take care of. I decided to hire Spirit Secretary and see how they did. I took the crazy cool idea to heart. For the next couple of months I didn't make long lists of the tasks I needed to do every day, instead I trusted that when I gave the task to Spirit, I would be reminded to do that thing in a timely manner. I was nicely surprised at the results. Driving down the road, I would see a license plate with the letters that reminded me of something that needed to be done. Sometimes, it was a thought that popped into my head. Other times, it was a passing image or an announcement over a loud speaker that reminded me of something that needed doing. The trust and connection to a higher source I called forth in the name of Spirit Secretary has served me beautifully over the years, although there have been times when I reprimanded Spirit (lightly) for not keeping me on track. Those are the times that I know I must reconnect with the Source. I have come to a balance between trusting in my Spirit and making lists, blended with the juice of mind mapping, I Ching and other spirit-physical connections.

Thank you Dear Friend,

for your support and kind love of my book. Together we form the Zing Living movement spreading Health and Yoga with Young Living essential oils and the Actions to make it all happen.

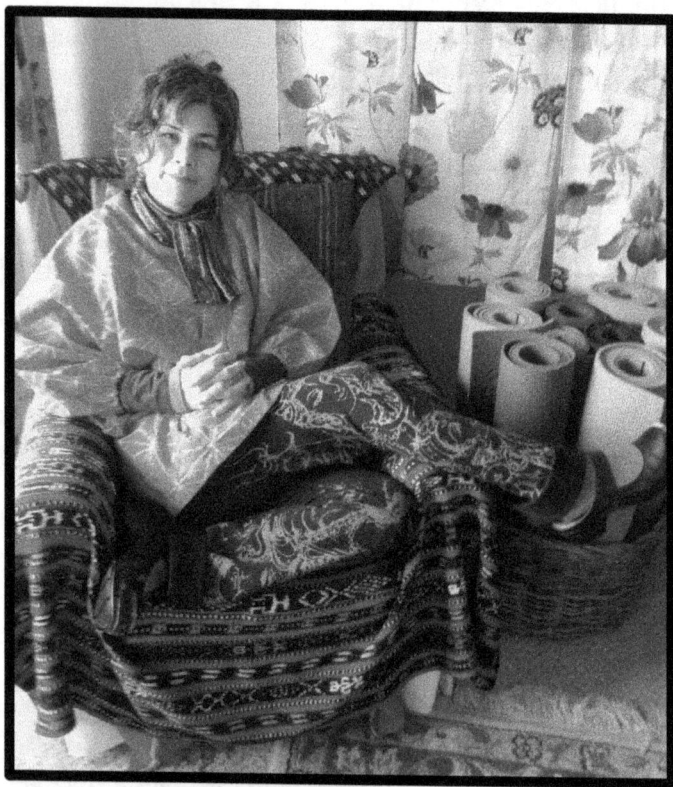

It's all about you loving yourself.

We are here to support you in creating the life of your dreams through books, videos and inspiration.
Keep moving in the directions of your dreams and believe in your magic.

Find us on social media:
@HeatherKamala
@myZingLiving
@KiDoKidsYoga
Our websites are the hub of information and sales:
www.myZingLiving.com
www.KiDoKidsYoga.com

Journaling for Health

After you complete the tasks in this book, be it weeks or years later (years in my case), return here to rate not only how you feel and look, but also how you now act, think and live. Then compare to your rating at the beginning of this book. Note where you can continue to grow, thrive and flourish.

On a Scale of 1 to 10, how do you rate your health? Circle one:

1   2   3   4   5   6   7   8   9   10

Write about all aspects of your health here.

Notes:

Notes:

Notes:

Notes:

Notes:

www.ingramcontent.com/pod-product-compliance
Lightning Source LLC
Chambersburg PA
CBHW050541280326
41933CB00011B/1671